I0709786

Perfect dog grooming tips

Beginner's guide to grooming your dog at home

Sharon K. Browder

Copyright©2022 Sharon K. Browder

All Rights Reserved

TABLE OF CONTENT

Introduction

CHAPTER 1: The benefit of dog grooming

Preventing dead skill and dirt

Prevent ear infection

Aid into detection of abnormality

Guard your dog joint and feet

CHAPTER 2: Keeping your dog clean and healthy

Wash your dog face

Take care of your dog nails

Bathing your dog with proper tools

Cleaning of the ear

Keep parasite at bay

Keep your dog arm and comfortable

Vaccinate your dog

CHAPTER 3: Feeding your dog and the procedure

Consult a veterinary nutritionist

Prepare simple meal for your dog Use enough amounts of essential nutrients

Learn how your dog nutrition vary with age

CHAPTER 4: introducing a heathy diet

Consider your dog mean

Integrate fresh vegetable

Increase your dog exercise schedule

CHAPTER5: Creating a bond with your dog

Participate in joint exercise

Hand feed your dog occasionally

Create time for cuddle

Maintain consistence communication

Periodically give them space

Build trust with your dog

Make time for fun and relaxation

Conclusion

INTRODUCTION

A dog's coat condition is typically a good indicator of how healthy they are.

Regular dog grooming may provide you with some early warning about potential health issues such as allergies, inadequate nutrition, parasites, or infections, or it may nip them in the bud.

Additionally, grooming makes you and your dog more sociable.

It also prevents the spread of diseases and fleas.

Self-grooming aids your bond with the dog as it helps the owner and the dog get acquainted with each other. This observation is borne out of my experience with my dogs so far.

Grooming can be a daily exercise. It all depends on the breed, age, and the dog 'state of health.

By using grooming products frequently, you can actually lessen the possibility that your pet will get unclean. A pet requires a lot of commitment to maintain. Dog owners should be careful to properly maintain and socialize their pets. Grooming is important, but also... additional material. A dog groomer must be able to make friends with pets because this is the only way to groom a dog successfully. You must know how to handle pets skilfully in order to complete all grooming sessions efficiently. Pets are very naughty and get irritated during grooming sessions, so you must master the art of pet handling.

A skilled dog groomer does grooming in such a way that the dog begins to enjoy the session rather than become angry.

One who is skilled at grooming dogs does it in such a manner that arouses the dog's love and confidence in its owner. Coat is like giving them a nice massage that promotes healthy blood circulation.

Grooming is a great activity for bonding. The more frequently you do it, the more accustomed you will become, and it should become a soothing, relaxing experience for you both. Too much grease can clog pores, causing irritation and other skin issues. Running a brush through their coat is like giving them a nice massage that promotes healthy blood circulation.

CHAPTER 1

The benefits of dog grooming

Even if your dog doesn't appear to be dirty, grooming provides numerous health benefits that may not be immediately apparent. Brushing your dog's coat helps it grow healthy and strong by removing old and damaged hair. Even if your dog doesn't appear to be dirty, grooming provides numerous health benefits that may not be immediately apparent. Brushing your dog's coat helps it grow healthy and strong by removing old and damaged hair. Additionally, grooming minimizes the amount of grease in your dog's coat and lets your dog's skin breathe. Too much grease can clog pores, causing irritation and other skin issues. Running a brush through there is a great activity for bonding. The more frequently you do it, the more accustomed you will become, and it should become a soothing, relaxing experience for you both.

When a dog sheds, the loose hair may become tangled and mat, which, if not frequently removed, can get worse and worse, dragging on the skin and leading to itchy, painful spots. If you aren't regularly checking your dog closely, it could go unnoticed.

It has been known to get so bad that large sores are produced, which can then become infected. All of this is concealed underneath their fur.

Dogs can't communicate their pain to us, so it's critical to maintain good grooming habits since it allows you to perform a basic wellness check on them. The area between their toes, where dirt and grass seeds can clump and collect,

should be inspected for matting and blisters. In addition to looking for any sores, fleas, or other general lumps, bumps, or scrapes, you can check their eyes, ears, and feet.

Preventing Dead Skin and Dirt

Dead skin and dirt will accumulate on your dog's coat if you don't groom them.

When you brush your dog, you assist keep their coat healthy and glossy as well as remove debris, dead skin, and dandruff from their coat.

The natural oils in your dog's fur are also stimulated when you brush their hair. As you brush your dog, these oils move throughout the fur as they are stimulated, this can make their coat appear shiny and healthy.

Additionally, brushing keeps your dog's hair from clumping or matting. Long-term matting of hair can cause skin rashes, bacterial development, and even parasite infestation.

You should brush your dog's hair every few days, regardless of the length of their coat. Wait until their fur is dry before attempting to brush them, and always brush in the direction of their fur.

When you brush your dog's hair after it has been damp, matting develops and becomes more difficult to remove. Additionally, brushes will cling to the damp hair and rip at the dog's skin, which could be painful. While several dogs like to be brushed, not all of them do. If your dog is immune to being brushed, there square measure some belongings you will do to create them a lot of cooperative. We suggest you begin by putting the comb ahead of your dog so that they will build friends with the tool. Once they've adjusted themselves with the comb,

reach out with it and gently bit it to their fur. If they permit you to the touch their fur with none resistance, reward them with <u>praise or a treat. Over time, you'll</u> <u>be able to increase the</u> pressure of your brush strokes.

Prevent Ear Infections

Ear infections can be avoided by regularly grooming your dog.

In particular, if your dog is prone to ear infections, you should clean their ears frequently. Dogs have a penchant for rubbing up against objects when they are out and about exploring.

This behaviour puts your dog at risk for ear infections and ear mites, both of which can be quite uncomfortable for them. They are even more susceptible to infection if your dog has particularly floppy ears. Wrap a cotton ball or pad around your index finger and use it to clean your dog's ears. Next, clean the exposed portion of their ear canal as well as their outer ear. Then, proceed to the other ear. Reward your dog.

Aids in the detection of abnormalities

The ability to keep track of what's happening with your dog's physique is one of the main advantages of grooming your dog. The more comfortable you become with the texture of their skin and physique, the more likely you are to notice something unusual. You'll be able to quickly identify any skin illnesses, underlying lumps or bumps, or patches by regularly grooming your dog. Early detection is crucial for all diseases, regardless of their type. Therefore, maintaining a healthy appearance will enable you to spot little issues before they turn into bigger ones.

Guard your dog's joints and feet

Grooming your dog additionally helps with joint and foot protection. So as to guard your dog's joints and feet, you wish to trim their nails on an everyday basis. If your dog's nails area unit too long, it'll force them to vary their gait that successively will build them come in a painful and unhealthy approach. Walking in associate unhealthy manner will eventually cause inflammatory disease and deformations. Beauty care is commonly the grooming step that dogs area unit most immune to Form your dog less immune to clipping, we recommend introducing them to nail clippers during a slow manner, as you'd with a brush. {|you'll be able to} begin by inserting nail clippers on the bottom and {so} inserting treats around them so your dog can inform itself with the thing. Eventually, you'll be able to bit the clipper to your dog's feet and, if they don't resist

Chapter 2

Keeping your dog clean and healthy

It's crucial to keep your dog clean for both hygiene and health reasons. Dogs that are well-kept are happier, healthier, and more enjoyable to be around.

Despite the significance of frequent washings, here are some more pointers and tactics to keep your dog in top condition.

Wash your dog's face

Due to their propensity for nose-to-nose contact, dogs are quickly contaminated in the mouth and face area. Due to the fact that dogs with wrinkled faces, such as Shar Pies', Pugs, and Drogue De Bordeaux's, will retain more filth and moisture there, it is crucial to maintain a regular face washing schedule. Dogs will not enjoy the shampoo stinging in their eyes, exactly as humans; therefore avoid the eye area while using a damp facecloth and a drop of dog shampoo. To maintain good hygiene, we advise bathing your dog's face three times a week at the very least.

Taking care of your dog's nails

Trimming your dog's nails at least once every month is something we advise. However, certain dogs' nails tend to grow more quickly than those of other dogs, so they could require more frequent nail trimming. If your pet's nails need to be trimmed, please contact the USPCA grooming room and our groomers will be happy to schedule your dog in. Cutting your pet's nails can be a little tricky and frequently results in some doggie drama.

Bathing your dog with proper tool

A bath doesn't have to be restricted to once each 6-8 weeks at the groomer. It's necessary to own regular baths reception permanently hygiene and to stay your dog's coat healthy. Dogs that pay longer inside could need less bathing than dogs that pay longer outdoors. we have a tendency to advocate laundry your dog no over once every week, it's essential that dogs aren't bathed too of times as a result of it will cause skin irritations, particularly if the skin isn't dried well or harsh soaps are used. Bear in mind to forever use dog shampoo. So, however does one

shut down once your dog? It's not like laundry automotive, unless your automotive likes to leap out of the drive once you're making an attempt to scrub it. First, you wish to create certain that your dog are able to fill in your tub on a plastic bath linen, or in a very plastic tub if you're doing it outside this can facilitate to confirm that your dog feels secure and isn't slippery around. Next, you wish to create certain that you're victimisation the right dog shampoo. Baby shampoo is best avoided as dogs have terribly delicate skin and even weak shampoo will cause irritation. For these reasons, we'd advocate solely victimisation dog shampoos so as to create your dog as safe and comfy as doable. Once your dog is totally soaked through, with water at an affordable temperature, apply the shampoo totally, however make certain to take care with the eyes and mouth and pay explicit attention to their hindquarters. Rinse and repeat, then totally dry your dog with a recent towel. whereas tub time are often difficult for each you and your dog, it's ultimately in their best interests, thus try and build it as calming or fun for them as you'll be able to, and you ought to haven't any issues laundry your dog.

Cleaning of the ears

Cleaning your dog's ears at least once a month will aid in infection prevention. They'll get the job done with a cotton pad and some warm water, and they might even like it! The safety of

your pet depends on your not using a cotton swab on your dog's teeth. How often do you brush the teeth of your dog? Daily brushing is recommended for your dog, but even two to three times a week will significantly improve their dental health. Use dog-specific toothpaste to avoid giving your pet any ingredients that could make them sick if they were to swallow human toothpaste. They should aim to brush their teeth as frequently as possible, ideally every day. It keeps their breath fresh and aids in the prevention of gum disease, which has been linked to other health issues such as heart disease and liver disease. Consult your veterinarian about the best dog toothpaste and toothbrushes. Additionally, keep an eye out for any signs of dental disease, such as bleeding, discoloured teeth, or extremely bad breath. During annual visits, your veterinarian should, of course, examine your dog's mouth.

Keep parasites at bay

Due to their natural curiosity, dogs frequently explore every inch of the yard, sniff everything in their path, lick objects of interest, and play with other neighbourhood pets. Due to their innate instincts, individuals unknowingly expose themselves to potentially dangerous substances, such as parasites. The best drugs for treating heartworm, flea, tick, and other parasites can be discussed with your veterinarian. These creatures can aggravate dogs and result in major health problems. Heartworms can cause lung disease and heart failure, fleas can cause anaemia, and ticks can transmit diseases like Lyme disease.

Keep your dog warm and comfortable

When the weather turns hot or cold, your dog requires extra assistance to remain safe and comfortable. When the weather is hot, take your dog for a walk in the shade or on the grass to avoid burning their paws on the hot pavement. Always provide them with plenty of water and shade. Ask your vet about a sunscreen you can use if they don't have much fur or have bald patches. Also, never leave your dog in a car during the summer; the temperature in a car can rise by 20 degrees in just 10minutes. The longer they stay trapped inside, the hotter it becomes. Even if it's only 80 degrees outside, a car can quickly reach 114 degrees. Exercise your dog regularly. Dogs, like humans, require physical activity. It maintains their weight and provides an outlet for their physical and mental energy.

This can help you control bad habits such as digging, barking, and chewing, which dogs are prone to when bored. What is the best form of exercise? Dogs crave human interaction, so plan activities that you can do together, such as fetch, walking, hiking, or swimming.

Vaccinate your dog

There are several alternative vaccinations that can protect your dog from deadly, easily treatable infections, even if state law mandates that all dogs be vaccinated against rabies. The immune system of a dog is better equipped to fight off any invasion from pathogens thanks to vaccinations. Antigens in vaccines imitate illness-causing organisms in a dog's immune system but don't actually cause illness. Puppies and dogs are vaccinated to help the immune system recognize the antigens present, which serves to slightly boost it. In this manner, if a dog is exposed to the actual sickness.

Chapter 3

Feeding your dog and the procedure

According to the saying, "You are what you eat," our meals provide our bodies with the nutrients they need for optimum performance.

The same regulations apply to your dog. Even though many dog owners are interested in feeding their dogs fresh, healthy meals to boost their health, you should first speak with a veterinary nutritionist. To stay healthy, dogs require a specific ratio of vitamins and minerals, and homemade dog food may be lacking in some of these nutrients. If you don't want to create meals for your pet, you may also purchase a selection of nutritious, naturally derived dog foods.

Consult a veterinary nutritionist

It is crucial to speak with your dog's veterinarian and ask for a recommendation nutritionist before you start cooking for your dog. You can create a nutritious diet for your dog and better understand his nutritional requirements with the aid of a veterinary nutritionist. Without first speaking to a veterinary nutritionist, never start preparing food for your dog. The wellbeing of your dog could be harmed by this. For instance, dogs who do not consume enough calcium phosphate in their diets are more likely to develop weak bones and teeth.

Prepare simple meals for your dog

There are a lot of quick and simple recipes you can use to make sure your dog receives all the nutrients it requires from safe, natural sources, despite the fact that this may seem time-consuming or complex. Before you start making meals for your dog, don't forget to consult a veterinary nutritionist. Making sure that your meals contain the right proportions of nutrients is crucial.

Depending on the age of your dog, change the food kind. You can require puppy chow or a dog food brand made for senior dogs if you have a puppy or an older dog. This age group of dogs has unique nutritional requirements that cannot be satisfied by standard dog food.

Use enough amounts of essential nutrients

Not every meal contains the perfect balance of nutrients, but we get what we need from a variety of sources or supplements over time. The nutritional requirements of your dog are the same. They may not get every vitamin they require from every meal, but if you understand what nutrients they require in what proportions, you can help them fulfil all of their nutritional requirements over time.

Learn how your dog's nutritional demands vary with age

In contrast to adult dogs, puppies require far more frequent feedings and must be given specially made puppy diets. The reverse is true for senior dogs, those that are seven years of age and older. They may just need one meal a day and will require much fewer calories. Dogs who are pregnant or breastfeeding may need to eat more calories, possibly more frequently. A low-calorie, high-protein meal served twice daily is recommended for adult dogs in general.

Chapter 4

Introducing a healthy diet to your dog

An initial examination of your dog with your eyes and hands might help you determine if your dog is overweight. Consider the shape of your dog's body from above. A small "hourglass" form should be discernible. Is your dog's belly (just behind the ribs) narrower than his or her front legs, chest, hips, and back legs? If this is the case, it is a good sign.

You shouldn't be able to detect any belly fat hanging down from your dog's tummy from the side. Can you lightly touch the last three ribs at the bottom of the rib cage? If this is the case, it is a good sign. It's time to schedule a visit with your veterinarian and start planning nutritional adjustments or looking for medical concerns that could be the source of the weight gain if your dog has obvious belly fat, you can't feel their ribs through the skin, or they don't appear to have an hourglass figure.

Together with your veterinarian, you can come up with a weight-loss strategy once you know what is best for your dog.

Consider your dog meal

The food you provide your dog can have an effect on their weight. If you feed a formula designed for active dogs or canine athletes to your inactive dog, you may be giving them more calories than they require. This would very certainly result in weight gain. Find a meal that is more suited to your pet's requirements.

A regular feeding schedule might help your dog avoid overeating.

Overeating can occur when your dog has constant access to food.

This is why we propose that our cuisine be served at specified times.

Integrate fresh vegetables

Boost your dog's food with some fresh fruit and vegetables. Green beans, carrots, broccoli, spinach, peas, cucumbers, melons, berries, and apples are just a few of the foods you can try to determine what your dog enjoys. To make sure your dog continues to feel full. Prior to serving, you might think about steaming them (except cucumbers; they can be served raw). Fruit and vegetables will typically add fibre and flavour to your dog's meals, but before including them in the mix, consult your veterinarian.

Increase your dog's exercise schedule

While it may appear that you may simply begin exercising your dog, you should develop a specific exercise routine. If your dog was previously inactive, you should gradually introduce him to exercise. Jumping right into a daily walking plan can result in joint pain or damage rather than weight loss.

Consult your veterinarian to determine the appropriate degree of activity for your dog. Consider some agility training as your dog tolerates more exercise. It's ideal for keeping your dog active and at a healthy weight. Because you have to work with them, it's also a terrific activity for bonding with your dog.

Remember to check with your vet before beginning an exercise regimen, just as we advise humans to do so. This is done to ensure that your dog is in good enough health to exercise. The activity shouldn't make any underlying medical conditions worse. Your veterinarian might advise you to start with a slight food change for your dog before adding exercise. Additionally, you might just want to begin with short, more frequent walks and work your way up to longer, more intense workouts. Sheltering in place? With these indoor activities, you can continue to stimulate your dog's mind and body.

When walking your dog, keep an eye out for any signs of pain, heavy breathing, or other discomfort. If you see anything unusual, make an appointment with your veterinarian.

If your dog eats dog treats or even foods like peanut butter or meat all day, it may be contributing to weight gain.

Delicious snacks should make up roughly 10% of your pet's diet. However, if you are taking obedience lessons or training for a canine sport such as Rally, Agility, or Fly ball, you may be utilizing treats as a reward to reinforce your dog's learning. This may result in a few additional treats, which shouldn't be a big deal if you adjust your pet's meals on the days you exercise accordingly. Increasing the duration, frequency, and intensity of your dog's walking routine will help him lose weight and improve his general health. You should probably include other activities to keep your dog engaged in exercise. Introduce one of the following workouts cycling or swimming once your dog is walking more comfortably.

CHAPTER 5

Creating a bond with your dog

There are always some particular things you can do to enhance the close bond between the two of you, regardless of whether you have a puppy or an older dog, or whether you have been dating for a day or 10 years.

Participate in joint exercise

Not only is exercise beneficial to you and your dog's health, but it can also help the two of you get closer. Going for a walk or a run is a terrific way to establish a joyful routine that allows your dog to experience new sights and smells while remaining by your side.

Hand-feed your dog occasionally

Hand feeding your dog treats a few times per week is another way to develop a special bond with your dog. Hand feeding your dog keeps their eyes and focus on you without much effort or persuasion on your part. While it takes more time than simply giving your dog food in a convenient bowl, it's a terrific way to bond with your dog and gain and keep your pet's attention.

Because your dog must be careful when eating from your hand, he is forced to concentrate on you and your directions. Your dog can establish trust and learn that you are his provider by rewarding positive behaviour with treats.

Make time for cuddles

Together, you and your dog should exercise in a healthy way, but it's also great to periodically relax. Spending time cuddling on the couch, in bed, or on the floor with your best buddy is a lovely, relaxing way to strengthen your relationship with your dog. Your dog may feel more secure and at ease as a result of physical touch, making him feels like a true member of your pack.

Maintain consistent communication

Do you generally desire you're not obtaining through to your dog? It's nearly such as you say one factor, however he hears one thing fully completely different. Which will be additional true than you think? during this article, you'll find out how to speak effectively along with your dog. Dogs area unit superb creatures. They adapt to innumerable things. Your relationship will be strengthened by having regular constructive communication. Make sure you're being consistent with your nonverbal cues and words when you're training your dog or just going about your They're extraordinary at associating, as well as learning the means or implication of the many sounds, like human language. A dog's "vocabulary" will reach upwards of one hundred fifty distinct words. But, despite however sensible, however skilful, and the way adjustable there, dogs can ne'er be verbal animals. Their tongue, thus to talk, isn't words however visual communication. Owing to this, it's solely natural that your dog can interpret your words through a "filter" — of visual communication, face expression, tone of voice, even your attention. And if one or additional of those "disagree" with the words you're mistreatment, most dogs can "obey" your visual communication. In my expertise as a dog trainer, most snags within the dog coaching method result from miscommunication, not fractiousness, stubbornness, or dominance. And whether or not your dog is strictly a family pet, a competition in canine sports, or full-time Canines familiars ,obtaining the foremost out of your coaching time suggests that learning to speak effectively along with your dog.

Possibly the primary factor to recollect concerning communication effectively along with your dog is that you just area unit taking a leadership role. Coaching your dog is, in fact, the final word expression of leadership; you're taking the initiative to show, guide, and direct.

Periodically give them space

Providing your dog with a private space will help you develop a stronger bond with him. Dogs are den creatures.

Create a place where your dog can hide out if he needs to take a break, such as a crate or a dog bed in a different room, in the event that he gets overwhelmed, wants to avoid noisy home guests, or just feels like taking a quiet nap.

It demonstrates to your dog how much you care and how crucial he is to you and the entire family that you take the time to be aware of all the things that can deepen your bond with him.

Build trust with your dog

When you're in the kitchen, teach your dog to sit or lie down on her mat. Treat her only while she is on her mat to thank her for making a wise decision. She'll figure out that she can have a treat while she's on her mat, but not when she's following you around when you're cooking.

Make time for fun and relaxation

Having fun together is another important aspect of creating strong friendships. Tug-of-war, chase, fetch, or "find it" games will strengthen your bond with your dog because you will be the centre of attention for all of his excitement. Don't be scared to be funny and have fun; she'll love your upbeat attitude.

Spending quality time with your dog will enhance your bond with her, so try doing it jointly if the weather permits. Spending extra time outside with you and your dog is always helpful.

Once they reach physical maturity, which occurs around the age of two years, many dogs make terrific running or jogging companions. This activity is ideal for keeping your dog entertained and busy while reducing boredom and releasing extra energy. Consider hiking, cycling, jogging, walking, and swimming, just to name a few activities

Participating in these pleasurable activities with your dog can help build your relationship. Involving your dog in your workout routine will strengthen her bond with you.

Conclusion

Cleaning is necessary for all pet. Grooming dogs is done for a variety of reasons. Pets require specialized care. A dog may only be appreciated if it is well cared for. Dog are affectionate. Grooming them might not be a big deal. Make sure to educate yourself on the breed of dog you on or are considering getting. The more you know about the breed and how to care for your dog, the more confident you will be in giving your dog a secure and happy home. Taking care of a dog may be an extremely gratifying experience because he will be a lovely and consistent companion. Be prepare to devote a significant amount of time and emotion to your dog.

www.ingramcontent.com/pod-product-compliance
Lightning Source LLC
Chambersburg PA
CBHW051701250726
48653CB00007B/2783